AL

DIET

Alkaline Diet: The Beginners Guide to Understand Ph,eat

Well and Quick Alkaline Diet Food List for Weight Loss and

Fight Chronic Disease

@ Joey Allen

Published By Adam Gilbin

@ Joey Allen

Alkaline Diet: The Beginners Guide to Understand Ph,eat

Well and Quick Alkaline Diet Food List for Weight Loss and

Fight Chronic Disease

All Right RESERVED

ISBN 978-1-990053-62-7

TABLE OF CONTENTS

Roasted Spiced Carrots

Ingredients:

For The Spiced Carrots:

- 1 teaspoon fennel seeds, toasted and ground
- 1/4 teaspoon salt
- 1 tablespoon sunflower oil
- 1 1/2 pounds carrots, peeled
- 1 teaspoon paprika
- 1 teaspoon cumin, toasted and ground

For The Tahini Sauce:

- 1/4 teaspoon salt
- A couple of tablespoons of water (until the sauce is a pourable consistency)
- 1 small garlic clove
- 1/4 cup tahini
- Juice from 1/2 of 1 lemon

For Assembly:

- 1/4 cup toasted pine nuts

- 1 cup of wild rice, cooked
- Alfalfa sprouts
- 1/4 cup toasted pumpkin seeds

Directions:

To Make The Spiced Carrots:

1. Preheat oven to 425°F and line a baking tray with parchment paper.
2. In a small bowl, mix together paprika, cumin, fennel seeds, salt, oil.
3. Toss carrots in spice/oil mixture.
4. Lay carrots in one layer on the baking tray.
5. Roast carrots for 20-25 minutes until the carrots are tender but still have a firm texture.

To Make The Tahini Sauce:

6. Mix all Ingredients: together in a food processor.

Alkaline Tempeh And Veggie Stir Fry

Ingredients:

- Asparagus, raw 3 spear, medium (5-1/4" to 7" long)
- Dandelion greens, raw 2 cup(s), chopped
- Garlic, raw 2 clove(s)
- Onions, raw 1/2 cup(s), chopped
- Liquid Aminos (Braggs) 1 1/2 tsp
- Olive Oil, extra virgin 1 tbsp(s)
- Tempeh, raw, firm 18 oz
- Carrots, baby, raw 3 oz
- Broccoli, flower clusters, raw 1 cup(s) flowerets
- Cauliflower, raw 1 cup(s)

Directions:

1. Clean vegetables and chop into stir fry sizes.
2. Slice tempeh into half inch cubes. Steam for 30 minutes than marinate for 20 minutes in tamari sauce or Braggs Liquid Aminos.

3. Heat oil and garlic and onions in a large skillet or wok over medium-high heat. Add the vegetables. Add tofu.

4. Add some Bragg Liquid Aminos which is a natural soy sauce alternative.

5. Cook, stirring constantly, 2-3 minutes, until tofu browns slightly. Add vegetables.

6. Stir for 1 minute, remove from heat and stir in teriyaki sauce. Serve with brown rice

Zucchini Tater Tots

Ingredients:

- Salt, pepper, and sweet paprika
- Olive oil
- 6-7 small potatoes
- 2 medium sized zucchinis

Directions:

1. Peel and cook the potatoes until they are fork-tender.
2. Let them cool down a bit until they are comfortable to hold.
3. In the meantime, grate the zucchinis and squeeze out the liquid with a kitchen towel.
4. Place the grated zucchinis in a medium sized bowl and grate the potatoes.
5. Add spices according to your taste and mix everything with your hands together.
6. Preheat the oven to 425°F and line a baking tray with parchment paper.

7. You might not fit all tater tots on one, so you may have to line a second one.

8. Use your hands to form small cylinders in the desired size and place them on the baking tray.

9. Brush each tater tot with some olive oil from both sides, so they don't stick to the parchment paper and bake for about 35-40 minutes, or until crispy.

10. Serve with desired dips.

Curry Roasted Cauliflower And Red Onion

Ingredients:

- 1 teaspoon turmeric powder
- 1 teaspoon garam masala
- 1/2 teaspoon salt
- 1/2 cup red onion, sliced
- 1/2 cup cilantro
- 1 head of cauliflower
- 2 tablespoons tahini
- 2 tablespoons water
- 1 teaspoon cumin seeds

Directions:

1. Preheat your oven to 400°F.
2. Cut the cauliflower into bite-sized pieces and place into a large mixing bowl.
3. Add the tahini and water to the cauliflower and mix well so that all the cauliflower is coated.

4. Doing this with clean hands is most effective.

5. Add the cumin seeds, turmeric, garam masala, salt, onion, and cilantro and mix well.

6. Spread the cauliflower in a single layer on a parchment-covered baking sheet and bake for 20 minutes.

7. Take out of the oven, flip with a spatula and bake for an additional 15 minutes.

Basil Pesto "Zoodle"

Ingredients:

- 1/4 tsp. cayenne pepper
- 1 tsp. sea salt
- 1 tsp. grapeseed oil
- 1/2 cup olive oil
- 1 key lime juice
- 1 lb. zucchini, in small strips
- 1/2 cup walnuts
- 1 cup cherry tomatoes
- 1 cup basil leaves

Directions:

1. Combine walnuts, tomatoes, basil, cayenne peppers, olive oil, and key lime juice in a food processor and process into a thick cream.

2. Sautée zucchini noodle with grapeseed oil until tender, but still crunchy, about 5 minutes

3. Add the pesto cream to the drained pasta and toss. If you find the cream too thick, add a little bit of water.
4. Serve with tomato halves.

Squash Casserole

Ingredients:

- 1 tbsp. coconut oil
- 1 tsp. dried rosemary
- ½ c. walnut milk
- 10 oz. butternut squash, peeled and cubed
- 1 tsp. salt
- 1 tsp. chili powder

Directions:

1. In a roasting pan, mix the squash with the other Ingredients:.
2. Preheat the oven to 375ºF.
3. Put the casserole in the oven and cook it for 40 minutes before serving.

Chickpea And Quinoa Fritters

Ingredients:

For The Fritters:

- 1 tsp. cayenne powder
- 1 of a key lemon, juiced
- 1/2 c. tahini
- 4 c. vegetable broth
- 1/2 c. chickpea flour
- 2 c. quinoa
- 2 tsp. ground tarragon
- 1/8 tsp. black bell pepper
- 1 tsp. salt
- 1/2 c.) chopped basil

For The Sauce:

- 1 key lemon, juiced
- 1/2 c. coconut milk
- 1/2 tsp. salt
- 1 tsp. chopped dill
- 3 tbsp. tahini

Directions:

1. Switch on the oven set it to 400°F, and let it preheat.

2. Take a medium pot, place it over medium-high heat, add quinoa, pour in vegetable broth, and bring it to a boil.

3. Switch heat to medium-low level and simmer the grains for 15 minutes until cooked, covering the pot.

4. When done, let grains cool for 10 minutes, fluff them with a fork, and transfer them into a large bowl.

5. Add remaining Ingredients: for the fritters in it and stir well until incorporated.

6. Shape the mixture into ten patties, arrange them on a baking sheet lined with aluminum foil and bake until golden brown and thoroughly cooked, turning halfway.

7. Meanwhile, prepare the yogurt sauce: take a medium bowl, place all the Ingredients: for it inside and whisk until combined.

8. Serve fritters with yogurt sauce.

Chickpea Fritters

Ingredients:

- 1 tsp. oregano.
- 1 tsp. dill
- 1 tsp. cayenne powder
- grapeseed oil
- 2 tsp. salt
- water as needed
- 2 c. chickpea flour
- 1 large white onion, peeled, diced
- 1 c. green peppers, diced
- 1 plum tomato, diced
- 1 c. kale
- 1 tsp. basil

Directions:

1. In a large bowl, mix all vegetables and seasonings, then mix in flour.
2. Slowly add water and mix, until the mixture can be formed into a patty.

3. Add oil to skillet and cook patties on medium-high heat for 2-3 minutes on each side.
4. Continue flipping until both sides are brown.
5. Serve fritters with alkaline flatbread.

Mushrooms Pilaf Fonio

Ingredients:

- 1 tsp. coconut oil
- 1 tsp salt
- 1/2 tsp. sesame seeds and black pepper
- 1/4 c. chopped onions
- 1/3 c. dry oyster mushrooms
- 1/2 c. fonio
- 1 c. vegan broth

Directions:

1. In a pot, sauté the onion, pepper, spices, and mushrooms in the coconut oil.
2. If the pot starts to get dry deglaze with a little bit of water till the onions become soft.
3. Add the water a little at a time using only what you need, sauce must not be too liquid.
4. When the onions are soft and translucent, add the veggie broth.
5. Cover the pot till the broth comes to a boil.

6. Let the pot sit for 10 minutes

7. After ten minutes, you can open the cover and fluff the fonio. Serve!

Fonio Porridge

Ingredients:

- pure agave syrup
- raisins (optional)
- 1 c. fonio.
- 2 c. walnuts milk

Directions:

1. Pour 1/2 cup of Fonio Grain into a medium-sized pot. Add raisins (optional).
2. Add milk and bring to a boil.
3. Turn down to medium-low heat and let simmer until liquid is absorbed (about 5 minutes).
4. Add pure agave syrup.
5. Stir from time to time to prevent the porridge from sticking to the bottom of the pot.
6. Leave to rest for 2 minutes, then serve.

Sesame Spelt Spaghetti

Ingredients:

- 1 tablespoon olive oil
- 1 tbsp. lime juice
- finely grated zest of ½ key lemon
- 1/2 tsp. dried chili flakes
- 1 tbsp. tarragon
- sea salt
- 7 oz. spelt spaghetti
- 4 onion, peeled, chopped
- 10 oz. chestnut mushrooms, sliced
- 2 tsp. sesame seeds
- 2 tsp. toasted sesame oil

Directions:

1. Put a large pan of water on to heat for the spaghetti.
2. Place the large pot over medium-low heat and add oil; when hot, add onion, salt and cook until softened.

3. Add the sliced mushrooms and cook them for 3–4 minutes over medium-high heat, turning them frequently in the pan.

4. Divide into bowls and sprinkle with the last bit of chopped tarragon.

Lemon Zoodles And Amaranth Greens

Ingredients:

- 1 c. amaranth greens
- 1/2 tsp. key lemon zest
- 1 tsp. olive oil
- 2 large zucchinis, trimmed and cut with a spiralizer
- 1 tbsp. key lemon juice
- 1 tbsp. walnut milk

Directions:

1. Put the zucchini zoodles in the bowl.
2. Add the rest of the Ingredients: and toss.
3. Then transfer them to the skillet and close the lid.
4. Cook on medium heat for 5 minutes

Ratatouille

Ingredients:

- 1 tsp. dried thyme
- 1 tsp. dried oregano
- 2 tbsps. avocado oil
- 1 tsp. salt
- 1 tsp. chili flakes
- 1/2 c. pumpkin, chopped
- 1 zucchini, chopped
- 1 c. cherry tomatoes, chopped
- 1 c. okra, chopped
- 1 red onion, chopped

Directions:

1. In the mixing bowl, mix up the chopped pumpkin, zucchini, tomatoes, okra, and onion
2. Shake the vegetables and sprinkle them with dried thyme, oregano, oil, and chili flakes.
3. Preheat the oven to 365ºF.
4. Line the baking tray with baking paper.

5. After this, put the vegetable mixture in the prepared tray and flatten it with the spatula's help and add salt to taste.

6. Cook the ratatouille for 30 minutes in the oven.

Spelt Soup And Mushrooms

Ingredients:

- 1 tbsp. cilantro, chopped
- 1 bay leaf
- 1 tsp. olive oil
- 4 oz. spelt
- 7 oz. mushrooms
- vegetable broth
- 1 tsp. salt

Directions:

1. Stir fry the chopped mushrooms and the bay leaf in the oil.

2. Heat for a few minutes and stir well.

3. Season to taste and remove the mushrooms from the pot.

4. In the same pot bring about half a liter of broth to a boil.

5. Rinse the spelt in running water and add it to the broth.

6. Cook according to the packaging Directions:.

7. Pour more broth if the soup gets too thick.

8. Ten minutes before the spelt is done, add the mushrooms.

9. Stir well and adjust with some salt.

10. Garnish with chopped parsley and a little raw olive oil. Serve hot.

Wild Rice Salad With Peaches And Radicchio

Ingredients:

- 1 cup chopped toasted walnuts
- 1 tsp. pepper
- 1 cup sliced dried or fresh peaches
- 2 tbs. watercress
- 1 c. wild rice
- 1 key lemon juice
- 1/2 c. olive oil
- 1 tsp. salt
- 1 head radicchio, chopped

Directions:

1. Cook rice according to package instructions. Let cool.
2. Make a dressing by whisking together key lemon juice, olive oil, salt, and pepper to taste.

3. When rice is cool, toss with remaining Ingredients: and dressing.
4. Serve at room temperature.

Baked Amaranth Patties

Ingredients:

- 2 c. vegetable broth
- 2 c. boiled garbanzo beans
- 1 tbsp. tomato sauce
- 1 tsp. chili powder
- 1 c. breadcrumbs
- 2 c. shredded zucchini
- 1 shredded onion
- 1 tsp. salt
- 1 c. amaranth seeds

Directions:

1. Preheat the oven to 400ºF.
2. Line a baking sheet with parchment paper and set it aside.
3. In a pot on the stove, place the amaranth and vegetable stock.

4. Bring to a boil, then reduce the heat to simmer, uncovered, until the water is absorbed.

5. Meanwhile, place garbanzo beans in a large bowl and smash with a potato masher or fork until mostly broken down (a few whole beans left are fine).

6. Add all remaining Ingredients: to the white beans, including the amaranth once it's cooked and cooled enough to handle. Mix well.

7. Form into patties and place onto the parchment-lined baking sheet.

8. Bake 20 minutes, flip the patties over, and bake another 10 minutes until crispy on both sides. Serve with a salad!

Garbanzo Beans-Spelt Cakes

Ingredients:

For The Cakes:

- 2 c. spelt flour, add more for dusting
- 7 c. of water
- 1 tbsp. salt
- 1 bay leaf

For The Stuffing:

- 4 oz. mushrooms
- 2 tbsps. olive oil
- 3⁄4 c. dried garbanzo beans, cooked.
- Coconut oil for the pan, frying
- Salt and freshly ground black pepper
- 1 medium onion, chopped

Directions:

1. Combine the water, mushrooms, and bay leaf in a large pot and boil a bit until the mushrooms are cooked.

2. Put the mushrooms in a bowl.

31

3. Add the spelt flour, stir to make the dough.

4. Add more spelt flour if the dough feels too sticky.

5. For the stuffing, add olive oil to a sauté pan and place over medium-high heat.

6. Add in onions and cook as you stir for 5 minutes

7. Add in the garbanzo beans together with pepper and salt (to taste) and cook for 2 minutes. Set aside.

8. To make the cakes, scoop about 3 tbsps. of the dough on your hand and press it into your palm.

9. Add a spoonful of stuffing on top of the dough and fold it over to close it.

10. Shape it into a round disk.

11. Now add coconut oil to a skillet and heat over medium heat.

12. Cook the garbanzo beans cakes on both sides until golden, roughly 4 minutes per side.

Sesame Ginger Rice Bowl

Ingredients:

- 2 scallions are finely chopped
- 1 bunch of cilantro, finely chopped (½ c.)
- 2 tbsps. minced fresh ginger
- 2 tbsps. sesame seeds
- 1 c. wild rice
- 1 avocado
- 1 cucumber
- 2 tbsps. toasted sesame oil
- 1 tsp. sea salt

Directions:

1. Cook rice as per the package's instructions. When done, transfer it to a bowl.
2. Top the rice with roughly chopped cucumber, avocado, and sliced scallions; garnish with sesame seeds.
3. In a small bowl, mix sesame oil, cilantro, salt, and ginger until well blended.

4. Then drizzle it over your rice bowl. Serve and Enjoy!

Amaranth Greens With Chickpeas And Lemon

Ingredients:

- 1 large onion thinly sliced
- 1 tbsp. grated ginger
- 1 key lemon zested and freshly juiced
- 1-ounce amaranth green
- 1 tsp. crushed red pepper flakes
- 3 tbsps. extra-virgin olive oil
- Sea salt to taste
- 1 can grape tomatoes
- 1 c. cooked chickpeas (rinse well)

Directions:

1. Pour the olive oil into a large skillet and add in the onion.

2. Cook for about 5 minutes until the onion starts to brown.

3. Add in the ginger, lemon zest, tomatoes, and red pepper flakes, and cook for 3–4 minutes

4. Toss in the chickpeas (drained) and cook for an additional 3–4 minutes.

5. Now add the amaranth greens in 2 batches, and once it starts to wilt, season with some sea salt and key lemon juice.

6. Cook for 2 minutes and serve!

Alkaline Electric Meatloaf

Ingredients:

- 1 tsp. Agave
- 2 tbsp. Onion powder
- 1 tbsp. Sea salt
- 1 tbsp. Basil
- 1 tsp. Oregano
- 2 tsp. Savory
- 1 tsp. powdered ginger
- 1/2 tsp. Cayenne Powder
- 3 cups Mushrooms, sliced
- 2 cups Cooked Garbanzo Beans
- 2/3 cup Alkaline Barbecue Sauce or Alkaline Ketchup
- 1 1/2 cup Garbanzo Bean Flour
- 1 cup White Onions, chopped
- 1 cup Green Peppers, chopped

- 1 Roma tomato, chopped

Directions:

1. Blend mushrooms and garbanzo beans together for 30 seconds in food processor.
2. Process for 1 minute or until fully blended in seasonings, agave, 1/2 cup of white onions, 1/2 cup of green peppers and 1/3 cup barbecue sauce.
3. In a large bowl, add the mixture and mix in 1/3 cup of onions, 1/3 cup of peppers and 1 cup of flour.
4. If the mixture is too moist put more flour.
5. Bake in oven for 35-45 minutes at 350 F.
6. Allow at least 30 minutes to cool before cutting into meatloaf or it may be mushy and fall apart.
7. Enjoy your Electric Alkaline meatloaf

Alkaline Electric Burro Mashed "Potatoes"

Ingredients:

- 2 tsp. Powder onion
- 2 tsp. Sea Salt
- 1/4 cup Green Onions, diced with Alkaline Gravy (Optional)
- 6-8 Green Burro Bananas or 2 cups Cooked Garbanzo Beans
- 1 cup Hemp Milk or Walnut Milk

Directions:

1. Split off the ends of each burro, cut each side through the skin, extract the flesh and add to the processor.
2. Pour the milk and seasonings into the food processor and blend for 1-2 minutes, then add spring water if the mixture becomes too thick.
3. Add mixture and green onions to a pan, and cook over medium heat.

4. Cook while stirring continuously for 25-30 minutes, adding more water when it becomes too dense. Serve, with Alkaline Gravy!

Alkaline Electric Mushroom & Onion Gravy

Ingredients:

- 2 tbs. Grapeseed Oil
- 1 tsp. Sea Salt
- 1/2 tsp. Thyme
- 1 tsp. Onion Powder
- 1/2 tsp. Oregano
- 2 - 3 cups Spring Water
- 1/2 cup Mushrooms (optional)
- 1/2 cup Onions
- 1/4 tsp. Cayenne
- 3 tbs. Garbanzo bean flour

Directions:

1. Add grapeseed oil over medium to high heat to fry pan.
2. Sauté mushrooms & onions for A minute.

3. Add all seasonings and spices except cayenne. Sautee for Five minutes.

4. Add 2 cups of spring water.

5. Add ground cayenne. Mix all Ingredients: completely and bring to a boil.

6. Continue sifting a little at a time the flour, and mix with a whisk to avoid lumps.

7. Start cooking until boiling, including remaining water if needed

Alkaline Electric Spicy Kale

Ingredients:

- 1 tsp. Crushed Red Pepper
- 1/4 tsp. Sea Salt
- Alkaline "Garlic" Oil or Grape Seed Oil
- 1 bunch of Kale
- 1/4 cup Onion, diced
- 1/4 cup Red Pepper, diced

Directions:

1. Rinse off the kale, then fold in half per leaf, then cut off the base. Air dry the kale.

2. Chop the kale into bite-sized bits and use salad spinner to drain water.

3. Add approx. 2 tbsp. Oil to wok over high heat.

4. Stir in onions and peppers for 2-3 minutes.

5. Reduce heat to low, add the kale to the wok and cover for 5 minutes with a lid.

6. Add crushed red pepper, mix and cover with lid for an additional 3 minutes or until tender.

Veggie Kabobs

Ingredients:

For Marinade:

- 2 teaspoons fresh oregano, minced
- 1 teaspoon cayenne powder
- Sea salt, as required
- 2 tablespoons fresh key lime juice
- 2 tablespoons avocado oil
- 2 garlic cloves, minced
- 2 teaspoons fresh basil, minced

For Veggies:

- 1 yellow bell pepper, seeded and cubed
- 1 red bell pepper, seeded and cubed
- 2 large zucchinis, cut into thick slices
- 8 large button mushrooms, quartered

Directions:

1. Mix all the Ingredients: in a bowl.

2. Mix in the vegetables and toss it well for evenly coat.

3. Cover and refrigerate to marinate for at least 6-8 hours.

4. Preheat the grill to medium-high heat.

5. Generously, grease the grill grate.

6. Remove the vegetables from the bowl and thread onto pre-soaked wooden skewers.

7. Grill for about 8-10 minutes or until done completely, flipping occasionally.

Spiced Okra

Ingredients:

- 1 teaspoon ground cumin
- 1 teaspoon cayenne powder
- Sea salt, as required
- 1 tablespoon avocado oil
- 2 pound okra pods, 2-inch pieces

Directions:

1. Cook the oil over medium heat and stir fry the okra for about 2 minutes.
2. Reduce the heat to low and cook covered for about 6-8 minutes stirring occasionally.
3. Add the cumin, cayenne powder and salt and stir to combine.
4. Increase the heat to medium and cook uncovered for about 2-3 minutes more. Remove from the heat and serve hot.

Mushroom Curry

Ingredients:

- 4 cups fresh button mushrooms, sliced
- 2 cups spring water
- 1/2 cup unsweetened coconut milk
- Sea salt, as required
- 2 cups plum tomatoes, chopped
- 2 tablespoons grapeseed oil
- 1 small onion, chopped finely
- 1/2 teaspoon cayenne powder

Directions:

1. In a food processor, add the tomatoes and pulse until a smooth paste form.
2. In a pan, heat the oil over medium heat and sauté the onion for about 5-6 minutes.
3. Add the tomato paste and cook for about 5 minutes.
4. Stir in the mushrooms, water and coconut milk and bring to a boil.

5. Cook for about 10-12 minutes, stirring occasionally.
6. Season it well and remove from the heat. Serve hot.

Bell Peppers & Zucchini Stir Fry

Ingredients:

- 1 large yellow bell pepper
- 2 cups zucchini, sliced
- 1/2 cup spring water
- Sea salt, as required
- Cayenne powder, as required
- 2 tablespoons avocado oil
- 1 large onion, cubed
- 4 garlic cloves, minced
- 1 large green bell pepper
- 1 large red bell pepper

Directions:

1. Cook the oil over medium heat and sauté the onion and garlic for about 4-5 minutes.
2. Add the vegetables and stir fry for about 4-5 minutes.
3. Add the water and stir fry for about 3-4 minutes more. Serve hot.

Barred Zucchini Hummus Wrap

Ingredients:

- 1 teaspoon cayenne pepper
- 2 tablespoons grapeseed oil
- 4 spelt flour tortillas
- 8 tablespoons hummus, homemade
- 1 of medium red onion; peeled, sliced
- 2 medium plum tomato, sliced
- 2 cups romaine lettuce, chopped
- 2 large zucchinis
- 1 teaspoon sea salt

Directions:

1. Rinse the zucchinis, cut their ends, and then cut into slices.

2. Take a grill pan, place it over medium heat, grease the pan generously with oil, and let it heat.

3. Meanwhile, take a medium bowl, place zucchini slices in it, season with salt and

cayenne pepper, pour in the oil, and then toss until well coated.

4. Spread the zucchini slices onto the heated grill pan, cook for 3 minutes until golden-brown, then turn the zucchini slices and continue cooking for another 2 minutes.

5. Set aside until needed.

6. Heat the tortillas: place them onto the grill pan and then cook for 1 minute per side until hot and grill marks appear on the bread.

7. Assemble the wraps: working on one wrap at a time, spread 2 tablespoons of hummus on one side of a tortilla, spread one-fourth of the zucchini slices, and then top with 1 cup lettuce and one-fourth of the tomato slices.

8. Wrap tightly, repeat with the remaining tortillas, and then serve

Vegetable Tacos

Ingredients:

- 2/3 teaspoon habanero seasoning
- 2/3 teaspoon cayenne pepper
- 1 key lime, juiced
- 2 tablespoons grapeseed oil
- 2 medium avocados; peeled, pitted, sliced
- 8 tortillas, corn-free
- 4 large Portobello mushrooms
- 2 medium red bell peppers; cored, sliced
- 4 medium green bell peppers; cored, sliced
- 2 medium white onion; peeled, sliced
- 2/3 teaspoon onion powder

Directions:

1. Prepare the mushrooms: remove their stems and gills, rinse them well, and then slice mushrooms into 1/3-inch-thick pieces.
2. Take a large skillet pan, place it over medium heat, add 1 tablespoon oil and when hot, add

onion and bell pepper and then cook for 2 minutes until tender-crisp.

3. Add sliced mushrooms, sprinkle with all the seasoning, stir until coated, and then continue cooking for 7–8 minutes until vegetables have softened.

4. Meanwhile, heat the tortillas until warm.

5. Assemble the tacos: spoon the cooked fajitas evenly into the center of each tortilla, top with avocado, and drizzle with lime juice.

6. Serve straight away.

Spicy Kale

Ingredients:

- 1/2 teaspoon sea salt
- 1 teaspoon crushed red pepper
- 2 tablespoons grapeseed oil
- 1/2 cup white onion, diced
- 1 bunch of kale, fresh
- 1/2 cup red pepper, diced

Directions:

1. Prepare the kale: rinse it well, remove its stem, and then cut the leaves into bite-size pieces.
2. Drain well by using a salad spinner.
3. Take a large skillet pan, place it over high heat, add oil and when hot, add onion and red pepper, season with salt, and then cook for 3 minutes or until beginning to tender.

4. Switch heat to low, add kale leaves into the pan, stir until mixed, then cover the pan with a lid and continue cooking for 5 minutes.

5. Sprinkle red pepper over kale, toss until mixed, return lid over the pan, and cook for another 3 minutes until vegetables have become tender.

6. Serve straight away.

Zucchini Noodles With Avocado Sauce

Ingredients:

- 2 teaspoon salt
- 1 cup walnuts, chopped
- 8 tablespoons key lime juice
- 1 cup of water
- 4 large zucchinis, destemmed
- 4 avocados; pitted, peeled, sliced
- 4 cups basil leaves
- 48 cherry tomatoes, sliced

Directions:

1. Prepare zucchini: remove the ends of each zucchini and then make noodles by using a spiralizer or vegetable peeler. Set aside until needed.

2. Place avocado into a blender, add basil, salt, and nuts, pour in lime juice and water, and then pulse at high speed for 1–2 minutes until smooth sauce comes together.

3. Transfer zucchini noodles into a large bowl, pour in the blended sauce, add tomatoes, and then toss until well combined and noodles are coated with the sauce. Serve straight away.

Enoki Mushroom Pasta

Ingredients:

- 4 medium bell peppers; cored, sliced
- 2 cups cherry tomatoes
- 2 teaspoons sea salt
- 4 tablespoons coconut oil
- 2 packs of enoki mushrooms, about 400 grams total
- 8 round slices of butternut squash, fresh
- 3 medium white onions; peeled, sliced

Directions:

1. Prepare the squash: cut the squash into eight slices, peel them, and then remove seeds.
2. Take a large pot half full with water, place it over medium-high heat, bring it to a boil, and then add butternut squash.
3. Cook squash for 30 to 45 minutes until tender, pour out the excess cooking liquid, and then mash by using a fork.

4. Add onion, bell pepper, and mushrooms into the pot and then let it simmer for 15–20 minutes until tender.
5. Season with salt, then remove the pot from heat and let the mixture cool for 15 minutes.
6. Add coconut oil, wait until it melts, and then stir well.
7. Divide pasta evenly among four plates, top with cherry tomatoes, and then serve.

Tuna Bites

Ingredients:

- 1/2 teaspoon dried oregano
- 1/2 teaspoon ginger powder
- 1/2 teaspoon dried thyme
- 1/2 teaspoon sea salt
- 1/2 teaspoon cayenne powder
- 2 tablespoons coconut oil
- 2/3 sheet of nori
- 2 cups walnuts, chopped
- 4 key limes, juiced
- 2 Roma tomatoes
- 1/2 teaspoon onion powder

Directions:

1. Prepare the nori sheets: fold it into three equal folds and then cut along the first crease to remove one-third of the nori sheet.

2. Now fold the cut one-third of nori sheet in half, cut along the crease, lay these pieces on

top of each other, fold them in half, and then cut along the crease.

3. Repeat with the remaining nori sheet and place the pieces into a food processor.

4. Prepare the tomatoes: cut off the tops, and then cut each tomato into five equal pieces.

5. Add tomatoes into the food processor, add remaining Ingredients:, cover with the lid, and then pulse for 3–4 minutes until well mixed and thoroughly blended.

6. Shape the mixture into rough balls, transfer them to a plate, and then serve.

Juicy Portobello Burgers

Ingredients:

- 4 teaspoons dried basil
- 2 teaspoons dried oregano
- 1 teaspoon onion powder
- 6 tablespoons olive oil
- 4 large Portobello mushroom caps
- 2 large avocados; pitted, peeled, flesh sliced
- 2 medium tomato, sliced
- 2 cups purslane
- Marinade
- 2 teaspoons cayenne pepper

Directions:

1. Prepare the mushrooms: slice it like a bun by removing the stem from each mushroom and then slice off 1-inch of the top.
2. Prepare the marinade: take a small bowl, place all of its Ingredients: in it, and then whisk until well combined.

3. Take a cookie sheet, line it with foil, grease it with oil, and then place the prepared mushroom caps on it.

4. Pour the prepared marinade into each mushroom cap and then let it rest for 10 minutes.

5. Meanwhile, preheat the oven to 425ºF.

6. After 10 minutes, place the mushroom caps into the oven and then bake for 10 minutes per side until tender.

7. When done, distribute baked mushroom caps among plates, cap-side up, and then stuff evenly with avocado, tomato, and purslane.

8. Serve straight away.

Chinese Cucumber Salad Magnifico

Ingredients:

- 3 tablespoon of sesame seed oil
- Just a pinch of salt
- Pinch of pepper
- 1 pound of fresh cucumber
- 4 cloves of garlic

Directions:

1. Take a bowl and add oil. Add salt and just a pinch of pepper.
2. Add minced up garlic to the bowl and toss them well to mix everything up
3. Wash the cucumbers well and cut them in half
4. Cut the halves into slices
5. Add the slices to the bowl and toss them well to ensure that they are coated well
6. Chill the salad in your fridge for 10 minutes

Buckwheat Pasta Mixed Up With Bell Pepper And Broccoli

Ingredients:

- 3 diced up middle sized tomatoes
- 3 sliced up carrots
- 1 tablespoon of fresh lemon juice
- 1 teaspoon of oregano
- 1 teaspoon of yeast free vegetable broth
- Sea salt as needed
- Pepper as needed
- 520 g of buckwheat pasta
- 4 tablespoon of extra virgin olive oil cold pressed out
- 2 diced up cloves of garlic
- 1 middle sized white onion ring
- Strips of 1 red bell pepper
- 1 big broccoli head cut up into florets

Directions:

1. The vegetables into bite sized portions.

2. Take a pot of water and add salt.

3. Heat it up and buckwheat pasta. Cook it to Al Dente

4. Take another pot and add broccoli and water.

5. Cook these as well. Take a pan and place it over medium heat.

6. Add 2 tablespoon of olive oil and add onions and garlic

7. Sauté them. Take out and keep it on the side

8. Add 2 tablespoon of oil to the pan and cook veggies until tender

9. Make sure to first cook the carrots, then bell pepper and finally tomatoes

10. Drain the cooked broccoli and add the broccoli and onions to the pan with vegetables

11. Add lemon juice, oregano, and vegetable broth

12. Season with salt and pepper to adjust the flavor. Stir well
13. Add the veggie mix over your buckwheat pasta and serve!

Chicken Salad With Almonds And Fruits

Ingredients:

- 1 can pineapple
- 2/3 cup dried cranberries
- 1 cup salted almonds
- 6 cups cooked chicken
- 1 cup mayonnaise
- 2 teaspoons curry powder
- 1 teaspoon salt

Directions:

1. In a large bowl, add salt and curry powder.
2. Whisk and then mix the pineapple, cranberries and chicken.
3. Transfer the mixture on a plastic covered round cake pan and refrigerate overnight.
4. The following day, remove the plastic cover and invert the cake pan on a plate.

5. Toss the Creamy Chicken Salad and garnish with chopped almonds and cranberries on top. Serve.

Blueberry Muffins

Ingredients:

- 1/2 cup almond milk
- 1/2 cup butter
- 1 tsp. vanilla
- 1/4 tsp. salt
- 1 cup applesauce
- 2 cups almond flour
- 2 tsps. baking powder
- 2 1/2 cups blueberries, fresh or frozen
- 1 cup granulated sugar

Toppings:

- 1/4 tsp. ground nutmeg
- 1 tbsp. honey

Directions:

1. Preheat oven to 375 degrees F.
2. Mix granulated honey and nutmeg in a small bowl. Mix well. Set aside.

3. Grease a muffin pan with 18 regular-sized cups or 12 large-sized cups

4. Cream butter using a wooden spoon or a rubber spatula in a bowl.

5. Add honey to the butter and continue creaming until fluffy.

6. Add one egg at applesauce.

7. Add salt, baking powder and vanilla.

8. Add half of milk and flour into the batter.

9. Fold and add the remaining flour and milk.

10. Continue folding until well blended.

11. Stir in blueberries. Fold to blend well.

12. Scoop the batter into muffin cups.

13. Top each muffin with a sprinkle of sugar-nutmeg topping.

14. Bake for 20 minutes until muffin is fluffy, moist and golden brown.

Pickled Mackerel On Cucumber Sandwich

Ingredients:

For The Sandwich:

- 1 lime, quartered, remove pips
- 2 Tbsp. apple cider vinegar
- 1 head red leaf lettuce, leaves separated
- 2 pieces cucumbers, halved lengthwise

For The Filling:

- 1 tsp. clarified butter
- 1 tsp. olive oil
- 1 tsp. capers in brine, drained well
- Dash white pepper
- sea salt, only if needed
- 1 jalapeño pepper, minced
- 4 Kalamata olives, pitted, minced
- 4 cherry or grape tomatoes, quartered
- 1 piece mackerel fillet, sliced into thin matchsticks

Directions:

1. Pour clarified butter and olive oil into saucepan set over medium heat.

2. Gently fry mackerel pieces until browned.

3. Transfer to plate and cover with aluminum foil.

4. In the same pan, add in tomatoes, capers and olives.

5. Stir-fry until tomatoes are a little wilted.

6. Turn off heat completely before adding in remaining Ingredients:. Stir.

7. Season according to personal preference.

8. Drizzle 1 tablespoon of apple cider vinegar on each cucumber half, cut side up.

9. Place equal amounts of shredded lettuce into cucumber cavities.

10. Add equal portions of warm mackerel on lettuce leaves.

11. This will wilt the vegetables a little.

12. Add in equal portions of tomato-capers mix.

13. Serve cucumber sandwich with lime quarters.

14. Squeeze juice on sandwich prior to eating.

Cobb Potato With Avocadoes

Ingredients:

- 12 small green onions

- 1 tablespoon lemon juice

- 3/4 teaspoon salt

- 4 ounces Blue cheese

- 1 olive oil-and-vinegar dressing

- 2 large avocados

- 3 pounds potatoes

- 3 large tomatoes

- 8 cups salad greens (mixed)

- Pepper

Directions:

1. In a deep-bottomed pot, add salt to boiling water and cook the potatoes for 30 minutes.

2. Once the potatoes are tender enough, peel the skin off, coat them with salt before slicing into cubes.

3. Pour 1 cup of olive oil-and-vinegar dressing over the potatoes and chill for 2 hours.

4. After 2 hours, prepare a plate and add the potatoes, green onions, mixed greens, avocado slices and lemon juice. Serve.

Mixed Greens Soup

Ingredients:

- 1 cucumber, chopped
- 1 zucchini, chopped
- 1 lemon, freshly juiced
- Pinch of kosher salt
- Pinch of white pepper
- 2 handfuls fresh spinach leaves
- 2 cupsmushroom stock
- 1/2 cup raw cashew nuts, soaked in water for 3 hours prior to us
- 1/2 cupfresh chives, minced
- 1 ripe avocado, flesh scooped

Directions:

1. Pour Ingredients: into blender; process until smooth. Taste; adjust seasoning, if needed.
2. Pour recommended portion into bowls.
3. This soup can be served immediately, chilled, or heated in microwave oven.

Crisp Radish Cucumber Arugula Salad

Ingredients:

- 3 Tbsp extra virgin olive oil
- 1 Tbsp minced fresh mint
- 3 small radishes, sliced
- Freshly ground black pepper
- 2 cups arugula
- 1/3 cup cubed cucumber
- 9 olives
- 3 Tbsp whole wheat croutons

Directions:

1. Mix together the mint and olive oil in a small bowl.
2. Season to taste with black pepper.
3. Place the arugula in a salad bowl and add the dressing. Toss well to coat.
4. Add the radishes and cucumber, then toss again to combine.
5. Top with croutons and olives.

6. Cover and refrigerate. Serve chilled.

Mushroom Hash

Ingredients:

- 1 cup thick coconut cream
- Pinch sea salt
- Pinch black pepper, add more if desired
- Handful fresh parsley, roughly chopped, for garnish, optional
- 10 cups button mushrooms, thinly sliced
- 1 cup water
- 2 Tbsp. wholegrain mustard
- 1 sweet orange, zested, juiced, pips removed

Directions:

1. Place mushrooms into the pan and cook these until seared on both sides.
2. Except for the bacon, add in remaining Ingredients: into the pan.
3. Stir and cook until sauce thickens, about 4 to 6 minutes. Season lightly.

4. To serve, divide mushroom hash into 4 equal portions.
5. Place equal portions into individual bowls.
6. Garnish with parsley if using. Serve warm.

Squash And Apple Soup

Ingredients:

- 1 cup non-dairy milk

- 2 teaspoon curry powder

- 1 teaspoon cumin

- Pinch of sea salt

- Pinch of black pepper

- 1 tablespoon olive oil

- 1 lb butternut squash, peeled

- 2 apples, diced

- 3 cups vegetable broth

- 2 teaspoon ginger, grated

Directions:

1. Set the oven to 375 degrees F.

2. Cut out a sheet of aluminum foil that is big enough to wrap the butternut squash.

3. Once wrapped, bake for 30 minutes.

4. Remove the wrapped butternut squash from the oven and set aside to cool.

5. Once cooled, remove the aluminum foil, remove the seeds, and peel.

6. Dice the butternut squash, then place in a food processor.

7. Add a non-dairy milk. Blend until smooth.

8. Transfer to a bowl and set aside.

9. Place a soup pot over medium flame and heat through.

10. Once hot, add the olive oil and swirl to coat.

11. Sauté the onion until tender, then add the diced apple, spices, and broth. Bring to a boil.

12. Once boiling, reduce to a simmer and let simmer for about 8 minutes.

13. Turn off the heat and let cool slightly.

14. Once cooled, pour the mixture into the food processor and blend until smooth.

15. Pour the pureed apple mixture back into the pot, then stir in the butternut squash mixture.

16. Mix well, then reheat to a simmer over medium flame.

17. Season to taste with salt and pepper.

18. Serve right away or pack for lunch on-the-go.

Banana Pecans Muffins

Ingredients:

- 3/4 cup butter, unsalted, melted and cooled
- 1 tsp. vanilla extract
- 1/2 tsp. salt
- 1 1/2 tsps. baking soda
- 4 bananas, overripe
- 2 cups almond flour
- 1 cup brown sugar
- 1 cup applesauce
- 1/2 cup pecans, chopped

Directions:

1. Preheat oven (375 degrees Fahrenheit)
2. Grease muffin cups on two muffin pans.
3. Combine flour, salt and baking soda in a large bowl.
4. Mix well by using a pastry blender or fork. Set aside.
5. Mash two bananas using a fork in a bowl.

6. Mix the remaining two bananas and sugar using a handheld or counter top electric mixer for 3 minutes.

7. Add vanilla, applesauce, and melted butter to the banana-sugar mixture. Beat well.

8. Scrape sides of the bowl to place the Ingredients: near to the mixing blade.

9. Add dry Ingredients: then blend.

10. Pour mashed bananas and pecans to the mixture.

11. Fold using a rubber spatula.

12. Scoop the batter into muffin cups. Fill each cup halfway.

13. Nudge the pan on the countertop to eliminate air bubbles.

14. Cook for 20 minutes or until cake tester or a barbecue stick comes out clean when the muffin is pierced.

15. Take the pan out to cool and serve at room temperature or warm.

Nutty Brussels Sprout

Ingredients:

- 1 teaspoon red pepper flakes, crushed
- Sea salt and freshly ground black pepper, to taste
- 1 tablespoon fresh lemon juice
- 1 tablespoon pine nuts
- 1 pound Brussels sprouts, trimmed and halved
- 1 tablespoon olive oil
- 2 garlic cloves, minced

Directions:

1. In A Large Pan Of The Boiling Water, Arrange A Steamer Basket.
2. Place The Asparagus In Steamer Basket And Steam, Covered For About 6-8 Minutes.
3. Drain The Asparagus Well.

4. In A Large Skillet, Heat The Oil Over Medium Heat And Sauté The Garlic And Red Pepper Flakes For About 30-40 Seconds.

5. Stir In The Brussels Sprouts, Salt And Black Pepper And Sauté For About 4-5 Minutes.

6. Stir In The Lemon Juice And Sauté For About 1 Minute More.

7. Stir In The Pine Nuts And Remove From The Heat. Serve hot.

Broccoli With Kale

Ingredients:

- 1 teaspoon fresh ginger root, peeled and minced
- 1 cup broccoli florets
- 2 cups fresh kale, tough ribs removed and chopped
- 1 cup coconut cream
- 1/2 teaspoon red pepper flakes, crushed
- 1 teaspoon fresh parsley, chopped finely
- 3 tablespoons coconut oil, divided
- 1/2 of small yellow onion, chopped
- 1 teaspoon garlic, minced

Directions:

1. In A Large Skillet, Melt 2 Tablespoons Of The Coconut Oil Over Medium-High Heat And Sauté The Onion For About 3-4 Minutes.

2. Add The Garlic And Ginger And Sauté For About 1 Minute.

3. Add The Broccoli And Stir To Combine Well.

4. Immediately, Reduce The Heat To Medium-Low And Cook For About 2-3 Minutes, Stirring Continuously.

5. Stir In The Kale And Cook Or About 3 Minutes, Stirring Frequently.

6. Add The Coconut Cream And Remaining Coconut Oil And Stir Until Smooth.

7. Stir In The Red Pepper Flakes And Simmer For About 5-10 Minutes, Stirring Occasionally Or Until The Desired Thickness Of The Curry.

8. Remove from the heat and serve hot with the topping of parsley.

Parsley Mushrooms

Ingredients:

- 12 ounces fresh mushrooms, sliced
- 1 tablespoon fresh parsley, chopped
- Sea salt and freshly ground black pepper, to taste
- 2 tablespoons olive oil
- 2-3 tablespoons onion, minced
- 1 teaspoon garlic, minced

Directions:

1. In A Skillet, Heat The Oil Over Medium Heat And Sauté The Onion And Garlic For 2-3 Minutes.
2. Add The Mushrooms And Cook For 8-10 Minutes Or Until Desired Doneness, Stirring Frequently.
3. Stir In The Parsley Salt And Black Pepper And Remove From The Heat.
4. Serve hot.

Garlicky Broccoli

Ingredients:

- 2 cups broccoli florets
- 2 tablespoons alkaline water
- Sea salt and freshly ground black pepper, to taste
- 1 tablespoon olive oil
- 2 garlic cloves, minced

Directions:

1. In A Large Skillet, Heat The Oil Over Medium Heat And Sauté The Garlic For About 1 Minute.
2. Add The Broccoli And Stir Fry For About 2 Minutes.
3. Stir In The Water, Salt And Black Pepper And Stir Fry For 4-5 Minutes.
4. Remove from the heat and serve hot.

Broccoli With Bell Pepper

Ingredients:

- 3 red bell peppers, seeded and sliced
- 1/2 cup homemade vegetable broth
- Sea salt and freshly ground black pepper, to taste
- 2 tablespoons olive oil
- 4 garlic cloves, minced
- 1 large white onion, sliced
- 2 cups small broccoli florets

Directions:

1. In A Large Skillet, Heat The Oil Over Medium Heat And Sauté The Garlic For About 1 Minute.
2. Add The Onion, Broccoli And Bell Peppers And Stir Fry For About 5 Minutes.
3. Add The Broth And Stir Fry For About 4 Minutes More.
4. Serve hot.

Spiced Okra

Ingredients:

- 1 teaspoon red chili powder
- 1 teaspoon ground coriander
- Sea salt and freshly ground black pepper, to taste
- 1 tablespoon olive oil
- 1 teaspoon cumin seeds
- 2 pound okra pods, trimmed and cut into 2-inch pieces

Directions:

1. In A Large Skillet, Heat The Oil Over Medium Heat And Sauté The Cumin Seeds For 30 Seconds.
2. Add The Okra And Stir Fry For 1-1½ Minutes.
3. Reduce The Heat To Low And Cook, Covered For 6-8 Minutes, Stirring Occasionally.
4. Uncover And Increase The Heat To Medium.

5. Stir In The Chili Powder And Coriander And Cook For 2-3 More Minutes.
6. Season With The Salt And Remove From Heat.
7. Serve hot.

Spicy Cauliflower

Ingredients:

- 1 jalapeño pepper, seeded and chopped
- 1 teaspoon ground cumin
- 1 teaspoon ground coriander
- 1 teaspoon cayenne pepper
- 1/2 teaspoon ground turmeric
- 3 cups cauliflower, chopped
- Sea salt and freshly ground black pepper, to taste
- 1 cup warm alkaline water
- 1/2 cup fresh parsley leaves, chopped
- 1/2 cup alkaline water
- 2 medium fresh tomatoes, chopped
- 2 tablespoons extra-virgin olive oil
- 1 small white onion, chopped
- 1 tablespoon fresh ginger root, peeled and minced
- 3 medium garlic cloves, minced

Directions:

1. In A Blender, Add ¼ Cup Of Water And Tomatoes And Pulse Until Pureed. Set Aside.

2. In A Large Skillet, Heat The Oil Over Medium Heat And Sauté The Onion For About 4-5 Minutes.

3. Add The Ginger, Garlic, Jalapeño Pepper And Spices And Sauté For About 1 Minute.

4. Add The Tomato Puree And Cauliflower And Cook For About 3-4 Minutes, Stirring Continuously.

5. Add The Warm Water And Bring To A Boil.

6. Reduce The Heat To Medium-Low And Simmer, Covered For About 8-10 Minutes Or Until Desired Doneness Of Cauliflower.

7. Remove from the heat and serve hot with the garnishing of parsley.

Eggplant Curry

Ingredients:

- Sea salt and freshly ground black pepper, to taste
- 1 medium tomato, chopped finely
- 1 large eggplant, cubed
- 1 cup unsweetened coconut milk
- 2 tablespoons fresh parsley, chopped
- 1 tablespoon coconut oil
- 1 medium onion, chopped finely
- 2 garlic cloves, minced
- 1 tablespoon fresh ginger root, peeled and minced
- 1 Serrano pepper, seeded and minced

Directions:

1. In A Large Skillet, Melt The Coconut Oil Over Medium Heat And Sauté The Onion For 8-9 Minutes.

2. Add The Garlic, Garlic, Serrano Pepper And Salt And Sauté For 1 Minute.
3. Add The Tomato And Cook For 3-4 Minutes, Crushing With The Back Of A Spoon.
4. Add The Eggplant And Salt And Cook For 1 Minute, Stirring Occasionally.
5. Stir In The Coconut Milk And Bring To A Gentle Boil.
6. Reduce The Heat To Medium-Low And Simmer, Covered For 15-20 Minutes Or Until Done Completely.
7. Remove from the heat and serve with the garnishing of parsley.

Lemony Kale With Scallions

Ingredients:

- 3 garlic cloves, minced
- 2 pounds fresh kale, tough ribs removed and chopped
- 1 cup scallions, chopped
- Sea salt and freshly ground black pepper, to taste
- 1 tablespoon extra-virgin olive oil
- 1 lemon, seeded and sliced thinly
- 1 white onion, sliced thinly

Directions:

1. In A Large Skillet, Heat The Oil Over Medium Heat And Cook The Lemon Slices For 5 Minutes.
2. With A Slotted Spoon, Remove The Lemon Slices From Skillet And Set Aside.
3. In The Same Skillet, Add The Onion And Garlic And Sauté For About 5 Minutes.

4. Add The Kale, Scallions, Salt, And Pepper And Cook For 8-10 Minutes.

5. Add The Lemon Slices And Mix Until Well Combined.

6. Remove from the heat and serve hot.

Veggies With Apple

Ingredients:

For Sauce:

- 1 cup fresh orange juice
- 1 tablespoon maple syrup
- 2 tablespoons tamari
- 2 tablespoons organic apple cider vinegar
- 3 small garlic cloves, minced
- 1 teaspoon fresh ginger root, peeled and minced
- 1 tablespoon fresh orange zest, grated finely

For Veggies & Apple:

- 1 cup red onion, chopped
- 2 apples, cored and sliced
- 1 tablespoon olive oil
- 2 cups carrot, peeled and julienned
- 1 head broccoli, cut into florets

Directions:

1. For Sauce: In A Large Bowl, Add All The Ingredients: And With A Wire Whisk, Beat Until Well Combined. Set Aside.

2. In A Large Skillet, Heat The Oil Over Medium-High Heat And Stir Fry The Carrot And Broccoli For About 4-5 Minutes.

3. Add The Onion And Stir Fry For About 4-5 Minutes.

4. Stir In Sauce And Cook For About 2-3 Minutes, Stirring Frequently.

5. Stir In The Apple Slices And Cook For About 2-3 Minutes.

6. Remove from the heat and serve hot.

Cabbage With Apple

Ingredients:

- 1 tablespoon fresh thyme, chopped
- 1 fresh red chili, chopped
- 1 tablespoon organic apple cider vinegar
- 2 teaspoons coconut oil
- 1 large apple, cored and sliced thinly
- 1 onion, sliced thinly
- 2 pounds cabbage, chopped finely

Directions:

1. In A Non-Stick Skillet, Melt 1 Teaspoon Of Coconut Oil Over Medium Heat And Stir Fry Apple For About 2-3 Minutes.
2. Transfer The Apple Into A Bowl.
3. In The Same Skillet, Melt 1 Teaspoon Of Coconut Oil Over Medium Heat And Sauté Onion For About 2-3 Minutes.
4. Add The Cabbage And Stir Fry For About 4-5 Minutes.

5. Add The Cooked Apple Slices, Thyme And Vinegar And Cook, Covered For About 1 Minute.

6. Remove from the heat and serve warm.

Herbed Asparagus

Ingredients:

- 1 teaspoon garlic, minced
- 1 tablespoon fresh parsley, chopped
- 1 teaspoon dried oregano
- Sea salt and freshly ground black pepper, to taste
- 1 pound fresh asparagus, ends removed
- 2 tablespoons olive oil
- 2 tablespoons fresh lemon juice
- 1 tablespoon organic apple cider vinegar

Directions:

1. Preheat The Oven To 400 Degrees F. Lightly Grease A Rimmed Baking Sheet.
2. In A Bowl, Add The Oil, Lemon Juice, Vinegar, Garlic, Herbs, Salt And Black Pepper And Beat Until Well Combined.
3. Arrange The Asparagus Onto The Prepared Baking Sheet In A Single Layer.

4. Top With Half Of The Herb Mixture And Toss To Coat.

5. Roast For About 8-10 Minutes.

6. Remove From The Oven And Transfer The Asparagus Onto A Platter.

7. Drizzle with the remaining herb mixture and serve immediately.

Veggie Kabobs

Ingredients:

For Marinade:

- 1 teaspoon cayenne pepper
- Sea salt and freshly ground black pepper, to taste
- 2 tablespoons fresh lemon juice
- 2 tablespoons olive oil
- 2 garlic cloves, minced
- 2 teaspoons fresh basil, minced
- 2 teaspoons fresh oregano, minced

For Veggies:

- 1 red bell pepper, seeded and cubed
- 1 orange bell pepper, seeded and cubed
- 1 green bell pepper, seeded and cubed
- 16 large button mushrooms, quartered
- 1 yellow bell pepper, seeded and cubed

Directions:

1. For Marinade: In A Large Bowl, Add All The Ingredients: And Mix Until Well Combined.

2. Add The Vegetables And Toss To Coat Well.

3. Cover The Bowl And Refrigerate To Marinate For At Least 6-8 Hours.

4. Preheat The Grill To Medium-High Heat. Generously, Grease The Grill Grate.

5. Remove The Vegetables From The Bowl And Thread Onto Pre-Soaked Wooden Skewers.

6. Place The Skewers Onto The Grill And Cook For About 8-10 Minutes Or Until Done Completely, Flipping Occasionally.

7. Remove from the grill and serve hot.

Tofu With Brussels Sprout

Ingredients:

- 1/3 cup pecans, toasted and chopped
- 1 tablespoon unsweetened applesauce
- 1/2 cup fresh parsley, chopped
- 1 pound Brussels sprouts, trimmed and cut into wide ribbons
- 1 tablespoon olive oil, divided
- 8 ounces extra-firm tofu, drained, pressed and cut into slices
- 2 garlic cloves, chopped

Directions:

1. In A Skillet, Heat 1 Tablespoon Of The Oil Over Medium Heat And Sauté The Tofu And For About 6-7 Minutes Or Until Golden Brown.

2. Add The Garlic And Pecans And Sauté For About 1 Minute.

3. Add The Applesauce And Cook For About 2 Minutes.

4. Stir In The Parsley And Remove From Heat.

5. With A Slotted Spoon, Transfer The Tofu Onto A Plate And Set Aside

6. In The Same Skillet, Heat The Remaining Oil Over Medium-High Heat And Cook The Brussels Sprouts For About 5 Minutes.

7. Stir In The Cooked Tofu And Remove From The Heat. Serve immediately.

Alkaline Electric Burro Mashed "Potatoes"

Ingredients:

- 2 tsp. Sea Salt
- 1/4 cup Green Onions, diced with Alkaline Gravy (Optional)
- 6-8 Green Burro Bananas or 2 cups Cooked Garbanzo Beans
- 1 cup Hemp Milk or Walnut Milk
- 2 tsp. Powder onion

Directions:

1. Split off the ends of each burro, cut each side through the skin, extract the flesh and add to the processor.
2. Pour the milk and seasonings into the food processor and blend for 1-2 minutes, then add spring water if the mixture becomes too thick.
3. Add mixture and green onions to a pan, and cook over medium heat.

112

4. Cook while stirring continuously for 25-30 minutes, adding more water when it becomes too dense. Serve, with Alkaline Gravy!

Alkaline Electric Mushroom & Onion Gravy

Ingredients:

- 2 tbs. Grapeseed Oil
- 1 tsp. Sea Salt
- 1/2 tsp. Thyme
- 1 tsp. Onion Powder
- 1/2 tsp. Oregano
- 2 - 3 cups Spring Water
- 1/2 cup Mushrooms (optional)
- 1/2 cup Onions
- 1/4 tsp. Cayenne
- 3 tbs. Garbanzo bean flour

Directions:

1. Add grapeseed oil over medium to high heat to fry pan.
2. Sauté mushrooms & onions for A minute.
3. Add all seasonings and spices except cayenne.

4. Sautee for Five minutes. Add 2 cups of spring water. Add ground cayenne.
5. Mix all Ingredients: completely and bring to a boil.
6. Continue sifting a little at a time the flour, and mix with a whisk to avoid lumps.
7. Start cooking until boiling, including remaining water if needed

Alkaline Electric Spicy Kale

Ingredients:

- 1/4 cup Red Pepper, diced
- 1 tsp. Crushed Red Pepper
- 1/4 tsp. Sea Salt
- Alkaline "Garlic" Oil or Grape Seed Oil
- 1 bunch of Kale
- 1/4 cup Onion, diced

Directions:

1. Rinse off the kale, then fold in half per leaf, then cut off the base. Air dry the kale.

2. Chop the kale into bite-sized bits and use salad spinner to drain water. Add approx. 2 tbsp.

3. Oil to wok over high heat. Stir in onions and peppers for 2-3 minutes.

4. Reduce heat to low, add the kale to the wok and cover for 5 minutes with a lid.

5. Add crushed red pepper, mix and cover with lid for an additional 3 minutes or until tender.

Veggie Kabobs

Ingredients:

For Marinade:

- 1 teaspoon cayenne powder
- Sea salt, as required
- 2 tablespoons fresh key lime juice
- 2 tablespoons avocado oil
- 2 garlic cloves, minced
- 2 teaspoons fresh basil, minced
- 2 teaspoons fresh oregano, minced

For Veggies:

- 1 yellow bell pepper, seeded and cubed
- 1 red bell pepper, seeded and cubed
- 2 large zucchinis, cut into thick slices
- 8 large button mushrooms, quartered

Directions:

For marinade:

1. Mix all the Ingredients: in a bowl.

2. Mix in the vegetables and toss it well for evenly coat.

3. Cover and refrigerate to marinate for at least 6-8 hours.

4. Preheat the grill to medium-high heat.

5. Generously, grease the grill grate.

6. Remove the vegetables from the bowl and thread onto pre-soaked wooden skewers.

7. Grill for about 8-10 minutes or until done completely, flipping occasionally.

Spiced Okra

Ingredients:

- 1 teaspoon ground cumin
- 1 teaspoon cayenne powder
- Sea salt, as required
- 1 tablespoon avocado oil
- 2 pound okra pods, 2-inch pieces

Directions:

1. Cook the oil over medium heat and stir fry the okra for about 2 minutes.
2. Reduce the heat to low and cook covered for about 6-8 minutes stirring occasionally.
3. Add the cumin, cayenne powder and salt and stir to combine.
4. Increase the heat to medium and cook uncovered for about 2-3 minutes more.
5. Remove from the heat and serve hot.

Mushroom Curry

Ingredients:

- 4 cups fresh button mushrooms, sliced
- 2 cups spring water
- 1/2 cup unsweetened coconut milk
- Sea salt, as required
- 2 cups plum tomatoes, chopped
- 2 tablespoons grapeseed oil
- 1 small onion, chopped finely
- 1/2 teaspoon cayenne powder

Directions:

1. In a food processor, add the tomatoes and pulse until a smooth paste form. In a pan, heat the oil over medium heat and sauté the onion for about 5-6 minutes.
2. Add the tomato paste and cook for about 5 minutes.
3. Stir in the mushrooms, water and coconut milk and bring to a boil.

4. Cook for about 10-12 minutes, stirring occasionally.
5. Season it well and remove from the heat. Serve hot.

Bell Peppers & Zucchini Stir Fry

Ingredients:

- 1 large yellow bell pepper
- 2 cups zucchini, sliced
- 1/2 cup spring water
- Sea salt, as required
- Cayenne powder, as required
- 2 tablespoons avocado oil
- 1 large onion, cubed
- 4 garlic cloves, minced
- 1 large green bell pepper
- 1 large red bell pepper

Directions:

1. Cook the oil over medium heat and sauté the onion and garlic for about 4-5 minutes.
2. Add the vegetables and stir fry for about 4-5 minutes.
3. Add the water and stir fry for about 3-4 minutes more. Serve hot.

Barred Zucchini Hummus Wrap

Ingredients:

- 1 teaspoon sea salt

- 1 teaspoon cayenne pepper

- 2 tablespoons grapeseed oil

- 4 spelt flour tortillas

- 8 tablespoons hummus, homemade

- 1 of medium red onion; peeled, sliced

- 2 medium plum tomato, sliced

- 2 cups romaine lettuce, chopped

- 2 large zucchinis

Directions:

1. Rinse the zucchinis, cut their ends, and then cut into slices.

2. Take a grill pan, place it over medium heat, grease the pan generously with oil, and let it heat.

3. Meanwhile, take a medium bowl, place zucchini slices in it, season with salt and

cayenne pepper, pour in the oil, and then toss until well coated.

4. Spread the zucchini slices onto the heated grill pan, cook for 3 minutes until golden-brown, then turn the zucchini slices and continue cooking for another 2 minutes.

5. Set aside until needed.

6. Heat the tortillas: place them onto the grill pan and then cook for 1 minute per side until hot and grill marks appear on the bread.

7. Assemble the wraps: working on one wrap at a time, spread 2 tablespoons of hummus on one side of a tortilla, spread one-fourth of the zucchini slices, and then top with 1 cup lettuce and one-fourth of the tomato slices.

8. Wrap tightly, repeat with the remaining tortillas, and then serve

Vegetable Tacos

Ingredients:

- 2/3 teaspoon habanero seasoning
- 2/3 teaspoon cayenne pepper
- 1 key lime, juiced
- 2 tablespoons grapeseed oil
- 2 medium avocados; peeled, pitted, sliced
- 8 tortillas, corn-free
- 4 large Portobello mushrooms
- 2 medium red bell peppers; cored, sliced
- 4 medium green bell peppers; cored, sliced
- 2 medium white onion; peeled, sliced
- 2/3 teaspoon onion powder

Directions:

1. Prepare the mushrooms: remove their stems and gills, rinse them well, and then slice mushrooms into 1/3-inch-thick pieces.

2. Take a large skillet pan, place it over medium heat, add 1 tablespoon oil and when hot, add

onion and bell pepper and then cook for 2 minutes until tender-crisp.

3. Add sliced mushrooms, sprinkle with all the seasoning, stir until coated, and then continue cooking for 7–8 minutes until vegetables have softened.

4. Meanwhile, heat the tortillas until warm.

5. Assemble the tacos: spoon the cooked fajitas evenly into the center of each tortilla, top with avocado, and drizzle with lime juice.

6. Serve straight away.

Spicy Kale

Ingredients:

- 1/2 cup red pepper, diced
- 1/2 teaspoon sea salt
- 1 teaspoon crushed red pepper
- 2 tablespoons grapeseed oil
- 1/2 cup white onion, diced
- 1 bunch of kale, fresh

Directions:

1. Prepare the kale: rinse it well, remove its stem, and then cut the leaves into bite-size pieces.
2. Drain well by using a salad spinner.
3. Take a large skillet pan, place it over high heat, add oil and when hot, add onion and red pepper, season with salt, and then cook for 3 minutes or until beginning to tender.

4. Switch heat to low, add kale leaves into the pan, stir until mixed, then cover the pan with a lid and continue cooking for 5 minutes.

5. Sprinkle red pepper over kale, toss until mixed, return lid over the pan, and cook for another 3 minutes until vegetables have become tender. Serve straight away.

Kale Wraps With Chili And Nopales

Ingredients:

- 1 tsp. fresh red chili, seeded and finely chopped
- 1 c. fresh cucumber sticks
- Fresh cilantro, finely chopped
- 1 c. cooked nopales
- 1 tbsp. fresh lime juice
- 1 tbsp. sesame seeds
- 2 large kale leaves
- 1 ripe avocado, pitted and sliced

Directions:

1. Spread kale leaves on a clean kitchen work surface.
2. Spread each chopped cilantro leaves on each leaf, position them around the end of the leaf, perpendicular to the edge.

3. Spread nopales equally on each leaf, at the edge of each plate, same as the cilantro leaves.
4. Do the same thing with the cucumber sticks.
5. Cut and share the chopped chili across each leaf and sprinkle it over the nopales.
6. Now, divide the avocado across each leaf, and spread it over chili, cilantro, and nopales.
7. Share the sesame seeds among each leaf and sprinkle them over other Ingredients:.
8. Divide the lime juice across each leaf and drizzle it over all other Ingredients:.
9. Now fold or roll up the kale leaves and wrap up all the Ingredients: within them.
10. You can serve with soy sauce!

Coconut Watercress Soup

Ingredients:

- 1 onion, diced
- 2 cup coconut milk
- 1 teaspoon coconut oil

Directions:

1. Preparing the Ingredients:.
2. Melt the coconut oil in a large pot over medium-high heat.
3. Add the onion and cook until soft, about 5 minutes, then add the peas and the water.
4. Cover and simmer for 5 minutes

Roasted Red Pepper And Butternut Squash Soup

Ingredients:

- 2 cups water, or vegetable broth
- Zest and juice of 1 lime
- 1 to 2 tablespoons tahini
- Pinch cayenne pepper
- 1 teaspoon ground coriander
- 1 teaspoon ground cumin
- Toasted squash seeds (optional)
- 1 small butternut squash
- 1 tablespoon olive oil
- 1 teaspoon sea salt
- 2 red bell peppers
- 1 yellow onion
- 1 head garlic

Directions:

1. Preparing the Ingredients:.
2. Preheat the oven to 350°f.

3. Prepare the squash for roasting by cutting it in half lengthwise, scooping out the seeds, and poking some holes in the flesh with a fork. Reserve the seeds if desired.

4. Rub a small amount of oil over the flesh and skin, then rub with a bit of sea salt and put the halves skin-side down in a large baking dish. Put it in the oven while you prepare the rest of the vegetables.

5. Prepare the peppers the same way, except they do not need to be poked.

6. Slice the onion in half and rub oil on the exposed faces. Slice the top off the head of garlic and rub oil on the exposed flesh.

7. After the squash has cooked for 20 minutes, add the peppers, onion, and garlic, and roast for another 20 minutes

8. Keep a close eye on them. When the vegetables are cooked, take them out and let

them cool before handling them. The squash will be very soft when poked with a fork.

9. Scoop the flesh out of the squash skin into a large pot (if you have an immersion blender) or into a blender.

10. Chope pepper roughly, remove the onion skin and chop the onion, and squeeze the garlic cloves out of the head, all into the pot or blender.

11. Add the water, the lime zest and juice, and the tahini.

12. Purée the soup, adding more water if you like, to your desired consistency.

13. Season with salt, cayenne, coriander, and cumin.

14. Serve garnished with toasted squash seeds (if using).

Tomato Pumpkin Soup

Ingredients:

- 1/2 tsp paprika
- 2 cups vegetable stock
- 1 tsp olive oil
- 1/2 tsp garlic, minced
- 2 cups pumpkin, diced
- 1/2 cup tomato, chopped
- 1/2 cup onion, chopped
- 1 1/2 tsp curry powder

Directions:

1. In a saucepan, add oil, garlic, and onion and sauté for 3 minutes over medium heat.
2. Add remaining Ingredients: into the saucepan and bring to boil.
3. Reduce heat and cover and simmer for 10 minutes
4. Puree the soup using a blender until smooth.
5. Stir well and serve warm.

Cauliflower Spinach Soup

Ingredients:

- 5 watercress, chopped
- 8 cups vegetable stock
- 1 lb. cauliflower, chopped
- Salt
- 1/2 cup unsweetened coconut milk
- 5 oz fresh spinach, chopped

Directions:

1. Add stock and cauliflower in a large saucepan and bring to boil over medium heat for 15 minutes
2. Add spinach and watercress and cook for another 10 minutes
3. Remove from heat and puree the soup using a blender until smooth.
4. Add coconut milk and stir well. Season with salt.
5. Stir well and serve hot.

Avocado Mint Soup

Ingredients:

- 20 fresh mint leaves
- 1 tbsp fresh lime juice
- 1/8 tsp salt
- 1 medium avocado, peeled, pitted, and cut into pieces
- 1 cup coconut milk
- 2 romaine lettuce leaves

Directions:

1. Add all Ingredients: into the blender and blend until smooth. The soup should be thick not as a puree.
2. Pour into the serving bowls and place them in the refrigerator for 10 minutes
3. Stir well and serve chilled.

Creamy Squash Soup

Ingredients:

- 1 tbsp curry powder
- 4 cups water
- 1 garlic clove
- 1 tsp kosher salt
- 3 cups butternut squash, chopped
- 2 cups unsweetened coconut milk
- 1 tbsp coconut oil
- 1 tsp dried onion flakes

Directions:

1. Add squash, coconut oil, onion flakes, curry powder, water, garlic, and salt into a large saucepan.
2. Bring to boil over high heat.
3. Turn heat to medium and simmer for 20 minutes
4. Puree the soup using a blender until smooth.

5. Return soup to the saucepan and stir in coconut milk and cook for 2 minutes
6. Stir well and serve hot.

Alkaline Carrot Soup With Fresh Mushrooms

Ingredients:

- 2 tbsp. olive oil (cold squeezed, additional virgin)
- 3 cups vegetable stock
- 2 tbsp. parsley, new and cleaved
- Salt and new white pepper
- 4 mid-sized carrots
- 4 mid-sized potatoes
- 10 enormous new mushrooms (champignons or chanterelles)
- 1/2 white onion

Directions:

1. Wash and strip carrots and potatoes and dice them.
2. Warm-up vegetable stock in a pot on medium heat.

3. Cook carrots and potatoes for around 15 minutes.

4. Meanwhile finely shape onion and braise them in a container with olive oil for around 3 minutes

5. Wash the mushrooms, slice them to the desired size, and add to the container, cooking for an additional of approximately 5 minutes, blending at times.

6. Blend carrots, vegetable stock, and potatoes, and put the substance of the skillet into the pot.

7. When nearly done, season with parsley, salt, and pepper and serve hot.

8. Appreciate this alkalizing soup!

Swiss Cauliflower-Emmental-Soup

Ingredients:

- 3 tbsp. Swiss Emmental cheddar, cubed
- 2 tbsp. new chives
- 1 tbsp. pumpkin seeds
- 1 touch of nutmeg and cayenne pepper
- 2 cups cauliflower pieces
- 1 cup potatoes, cubed
- 2 cups vegetable stock (without yeast)

Directions:

1. Cook cauliflower and potato in vegetable stock until delicate and blend them.
2. Season the soup with nutmeg and cayenne, and possibly somewhat salt and pepper.
3. Include cheddar and chives and mix a couple of moments until the soup is smooth and prepared to serve.
4. Enhance it with pumpkin seeds.

Chilled Avocado Tomato Soup

Ingredients:

- 1 clove of garlic
- Juice of 1 fresh lemon
- 1 cup of water (best: alkaline water)
- A handful of fresh lavages
- Parsley and sea salt to taste
- 2 small avocados
- 2 large tomatoes
- 1 stalk of celery
- 1 small onion

Directions:

1. Scoop the avocados and cut all veggies into little pieces.
2. Spot all fixings in a blender and blend until smooth.
3. Serve chilled and appreciate this nutritious and sound soluble soup formula!

Pumpkin And White Bean Soup With Sage

Ingredients:

- 1 tbsp. of cold squeezed additional virgin olive oil
- 1 tbsp. of spices (your top picks)
- 1 tbsp. of sage
- 2 quart water (best: antacid water)
- A spot of ocean salt and pepper
- 2 pound pumpkin
- 1 pound yams
- 1 pound white beans
- 1 onion
- 2 cloves of garlic

Directions:

1. Cut the pumpkin and potatoes in shapes, cut the onion, and cut the garlic, the spices, and the sage into fine pieces.

2. Sauté the onion and also the garlic in olive oil for around two or three minutes

3. Include the potatoes, pumpkin, spices, and sage and fry for an additional 5 minutes

4. At that point include the water and cook for around 30 minutes (spread the pot with a top) until vegetables are delicate.

5. At long last include the beans and some salt and pepper.

6. Cook for an additional 5 minutes and serve right away.

7. Prepared!! Appreciate this antacid soup. Alkalizing tasty!

Alkaline Carrot Soup With Millet

Ingredients:

- 2 tbsp. new chives
- 1 tbsp. pumpkin seeds
- 1 touch of nutmeg and cayenne pepper
- 2 cups cauliflower pieces
- 1 cup potatoes, cubed
- 2 cups vegetable stock (without yeast)
- 3 tbsp. Swiss Emmental cheddar, cubed

Directions:

1. Cook cauliflower and potato in vegetable stock until delicate and blend them.
2. Season the soup with nutmeg and cayenne, and possibly somewhat salt and pepper.
3. Include Emmental cheddar and chives and mix a couple of moments until the soup is smooth and prepared to serve.
4. It can be enhanced with pumpkin seeds.

Pumpkin Tomato Soup

Ingredients:

- 5 yellow onions
- 1 tbsp. cold squeezed additional virgin olive oil
- 2 tsp. ocean salt or natural salt
- Touch of cayenne pepper
- Your preferred spices (discretionary)
- Bunch of new parsley
- 1 quart of water (if accessible: soluble water)
- 420 g new tomatoes, stripped and diced
- 1 medium-sized sweet pumpkin

Directions:

1. Cut onions in little pieces and sauté with some oil in a significant pot.
2. Cut the pumpkin down the middle, at that point remove the stem and scoop out the seeds.

3. At long last scoop out the fragile living creature and put it in the pot.

4. Include likewise the tomatoes and the water and cook for around 20 minutes

5. At that point empty the soup into a food processor and blend well for a couple of moments.

6. Sprinkle with salt, pepper, and other spices.

7. Fill bowls and trimming with new parsley.

8. Make the most of your alkalizing soup!

Alkaline Pumpkin Coconut Soup

Ingredients:

- 3 ounces leek
- 1 bunch of new parsley
- 1 touch of nutmeg
- 1 touch of cayenne pepper
- 1 tsp. ocean salt or natural salt
- 4 tbsp. cold squeezed additional virgin olive oil
- 2lb pumpkin
- 6 cups of water (best: soluble water delivered with a water ionizer)
- 1 cup low-fat coconut milk
- 5 ounces of potatoes
- 2 major onions

Directions:

1. As a matter of first significance: cut the onions, the pumpkin, and the potatoes just as the hole into little pieces.

2. At that point, heat the olive oil in a significant pot and sauté the onions for a couple of moments.
3. At that point, include the water and heat the pumpkin, potatoes, and the leek until delicate.
4. Include coconut milk.
5. Presently utilize a hand blender and puree for around 1 moment.
6. The soup should turn out to be extremely velvety.
7. Season with salt, pepper, and nutmeg.
8. Lastly, include the parsley and appreciate this alkalizing pumpkin soup hot or cold.

Cold Cauliflower-Coconut Soup

Ingredients:

- 1/3 cup cold squeezed additional virgin olive oil
- 1 cup new coriander leaves, slashed
- Spot of salt and cayenne pepper
- 1 bunch of unsweetened coconut chips
- 1 pound (470 g) new cauliflower
- 2 cup (310 ml) unsweetened coconut milk
- 1 cup of water (best: antacid water)
- 2 tbsp. new lime juice

Directions:

1. Steam cauliflower for around 10 minutes
2. At that point, set up the cauliflower with coconut milk and water in a food processor and get it started until extremely smooth.
3. Include a new lime squeeze, salt and pepper, a large portion of the cleaved coriander, and

the oil and blend for an additional couple of moments.

4. Pour in soup bowls and embellishment with coriander and coconut chips. Enjoy!

Raw Avocado-Broccoli Soup With Cashew Nuts

Ingredients:

- 1 clove of garlic
- 1 tbsp. cold-pressed extra virgin olive oil
- 1 pinch of sea salt and pepper
- Some parsley to garnish
- 1 cup of water (if available: alkaline water)
- 1 avocado
- 1 cup chopped broccoli
- 1 cup cashew nuts
- 1 cup alfalfa sprouts

Directions:

1. Put the cashew nuts in a blender or food processor, include some water and puree for a couple of moments.

2. Include the various fixings (except for the avocado) individually and puree each an ideal opportunity for a couple of moments.

3. Dispense the soup in a container and warm it up to the normal room temperature.

4. Enhance with salt and pepper.

5. In the interim dice the avocado and slash the parsley.

6. Dispense the soup in a container or plate; include the avocado slices and embellishment with parsley.

7. That's it! Enjoy this excellent healthy soup!

Chilled Cucumber And Lime Soup

Ingredients:

- 1 tablespoon fresh cilantro leaves
- 1 garlic clove, crushed
- 1/2 teaspoon of sea salt
- 1 cucumber, peeled
- zucchini, peeled
- 1 tablespoon freshly squeezed lime juice

Directions:

1. In a blender, blend the cucumber, zucchini, lime juice, cilantro, garlic, and salt until well combined. Add more salt, if necessary.

2. Fill 1 huge or 2 little dishes and enjoy immediately or refrigerate for 15 to 20 minutes to chill before serving.

Lime & Mint Summer Fruit Salad

Ingredients:

- 1/2 cup peaches, peeled and diced
- 1/2 cup tangerine slices
- 1/2 cup cantaloupe, small bite-size pieces
- 1/2 cup honeydew melon, small bite-size pieces
- 1/2 cup watermelon, small bite-size pieces
- 1/2 cup apple, peeled and diced
- 1/2 cup grapes
- 2 tablespoons mint, fresh and chopped
- 2 tablespoons Seville orange juice, freshly squeezed
- 1/2 cup strawberries

Directions:

1. In a mixing bowl, combine all of the fruit.
2. Add the Seville orange juice, mint, and mix well.
3. Serve chilled and enjoy!

Cherry Tomato & Kale Salad

Ingredients:

- 2 cups organic baby tomatoes
- 1 bunch kale, stemmed, leaves washed and chopped
- 2 tbsps. Ranch dressing

Directions:

1. Mix all the Ingredients: in a bowl.
2. Divide the salad equally into two serving dishes.
3. Serve.

Radish Noodle Salad

Ingredients:

- 1 chopped scallion
- 1 tbsp. sesame oil
- 1 bell seeded pepper, cut into strips
- 2 tbsps. Toasted sesame seeds
- 1 tsp. sea salt
- 1 tsp. red pepper flakes
- 2 cups cooked radish florets
- 1 roasted spaghetti squash

Directions:

1. Start by preparing the spaghetti squash by removing the cooked squash with a fork into a bowl.
2. Add the radish, red bell pepper, and scallion to the bowl with the squash.
3. In a small bowl, mix the red pepper flakes, salt, and sesame oil.

4. Drizzle the mixture to top the vegetables. Toss gently to combine them.

5. Add the sesame seeds to garnish. Serve.

Caprese Salad

Ingredients:

- 1 bunch basil leaves
- 1 tsp. sea salt
- 1 cup cubed jackfruit
- 1 sliced avocado
- 2 sliced large tomatoes

Directions:

1. In a bowl toss all the salad Ingredients: to mix.
2. Add the sea salt to the season. Serve.

Summer Lettuce Salad

Ingredients:

- 1 peeled and sliced cucumber
- 2 thinly sliced radishes
- 1 sliced scallion
- 1/2 cup shredded zucchini
- 14 oz. can drain whole green beans
- 2 cups halved cherry tomatoes
- 4 cups romaine lettuce or iceberg

Directions:

1. Add all of the salad Ingredients: in a large bowl then toss with 2 tbsps. Of the dressing.
2. Serve.

Mustard Cabbage Salad

Ingredients:

- 2 tablespoons mustard
- 1 teaspoon hot paprika
- 1 tablespoon dill, chopped
- 1 green cabbage head, shredded
- 1 red cabbage head, shredded
- 2 tablespoons avocado oil

Directions:

1. In a bowl, mix the cabbage with the oil, mustard, and the other Ingredients:, toss, divide between plates and serve as a side salad.

Alkaline-Electric Spring Salad

Ingredients:

- 1/4 cup walnuts
- 1/4 cup approved herbs
- 1 cup cherry tomatoes
- 4 cups seasonal greens

For the dressing:

- 1 tablespoon of homemade raw sesame tahini butter
- Sea salt and cayenne pepper
- 3 key limes

Directions:

1. Sap the key limes.
2. Whisk together the homemade raw sesame "tahini" butter with the key lime juice in a small bowl.
3. Add cayenne pepper and sea salt to your satisfaction.
4. Cut the cherry tomatoes in half.

5. In a large bowl, combine the greens, cherry tomatoes, and herbs.

6. Pour the dressing on top and massage with your hands.

7. Let the greens soak the dressing.

8. Add more cayenne pepper, herbs, and sea salt.

Mix-Mix Alkaline Veggie

Ingredients:

- 5-10 sliced olives

- 1/2 red bell pepper (chopped)

- 1/2 green bell pepper (chopped)

- 1 tbsp. 100% date sugar syrup

- 3 tbsp. water

- 1 tsp of sea salt

- 15 kale leaves (chopped)

- 1 cup of watercress leaves

- 1 cucumber (diced)

- 2 tbsp. fresh dill (finely chopped)

- 1/ red onion (chopped)

Directions:

1. Mix the date sugar syrup, water, and salt together.

2. Stir in the remaining Ingredients: together in a bowl.

3. Massage in date syrup mix with the vegetables. Toss and serve.

Nori Wraps With Fresh Vegetables And Quinoa

Ingredients:

- 1bsp Raw seed mix
- 1tsp Fresh ginger root, finely grated
- cup Raw cucumber sticks/
- cup Fresh coriander leaves, finely chopped/
- 1 tbsp Sesame oilseed
- 2 Nori sheets
- cup Raw carrot sticks/
- cup Cooked quinoa
- cup Raw carrot sticks/
- 1tsp Fresh garlic, finely chopped

Directions:

1. Get a bowl and mix cooked quinoa with coriander leaves, ginger, seed mix, coriander leaves, and garlic.

2. Pour the sesame oil seed and mix properly.

3. Spread out both nori sheets on two surfaces.

4. Spread the quinoa mix one each nori sheets. Add carrot sticks and cucumber on top of the quinoa.

5. Fold up the nori sheets with the quinoa Ingredients: inside.

6. Depending on how you like it, serve with pickled ginger or soy sauce.

Kale Wraps With Chili, Garlic, Cucumber, Coriander, And Green Beans

Ingredients:

- 1 tsp Fresh red chili
- 1 cup Fresh cucumber sticks
- cup Fresh coriander leaves
- 1 cup Green beans
- 1 tbsp Fresh lime juice
- 1 tbsp Raw seed mix
- 2 Kale leaves
- 2 tsp Fresh garlic
- Ripe avocado

Directions:

1. Spread kale leaves on a clean kitchen work surface.
2. Spread each chopped coriander leaves on each leaf, position them around the end of the leaf, perpendicular to the edge.

3. Spread green beans equally on each leaf, at the edge of each leaf, same as the coriander leaves.
4. Do the same thing with the cucumber sticks.
5. Cut the divide chopped garlic across each leaf, sprinkling it all over the green beans.
6. Cut and share the chopped chili across each leaf and sprinkle it over the garlic.
7. Now, divide the avocado across each leaf, and spread it over chili, garlic, coriander and green beans.
8. Share the raw seed mix among each leaf, and sprinkle them over other Ingredients:.
9. Divide the lime juice on across each leaf and drizzle it over all other Ingredients:.
10. Now fold or roll up the kale leaves and wrap up all the Ingredients: within it.
11. You can serve with soy sauce!

Cabbage Wraps With Avocado, Asparagus, Pecan Nuts And Strawberries

Ingredients:

- 2 Cabbage leaves
- 1 Ripe avocado
- 1 cup Green asparagus spears
- cup Raw pecan nuts
- cup Fresh sliced strawberries

Directions:

1. Spread out the cabbage sheets on a clean kitchen work surface.
2. Share the asparagus shear among each cabbage leaf and place them on the edge of the leaf.
3. Share the avocado slices on each leaf and put them on top of the asparagus spears.
4. Share the strawberries over each leaf and spread on top of the avocado slices.

5. Share the pecan nuts between each leaf and spread it on the strawberries.

6. Wrap the leaves with all Ingredients: inside them. Serve with soy sauce (optional).

Millet Tabbouleh, Lime And Cilantro

Ingredients:

- 2 Tomatoes
- 2 Green onions
- 2 Cucumber
- 1 cup Millet
- 1 cup Lime juice
- 1 cup Cilantro
- 6 drops Hot sauce
- 1/2 cup and 2tsp Olive oil

Directions:

1. Heat olive oil in a saucepan over medium heat.
2. Add the millet and fry until it begins to smell fragrant (this takes between three (3) to four (4) minutes).
3. Add about six (6) cups of water and bring to boil.
4. Wait for about fifteen (15) minutes.

5. Turn off the heat, wash and rinse under cold water.

6. Drain the millet and transfer to a large bowl.

7. Add cucumbers, tomatoes, lime juice, cilantro, green onions, the 1/2 cup oil, and hot sauce.

8. Season with pepper and salt to taste.

Alkaline Cauliflower Fried Rice With Kale, Ginger, And Turmeric

Ingredients:

- 1 Zucchini (courgette)
- 1 bunch Kale
- 1 Cauliflower
- 1 tsp Tamari soy sauce
- 1 bunch Parsley
- 1 Lime
- 4 Spring onions
- 2 Almonds
- 1 tbsp Coconut oil
- 1 Cauliflower (large
- 1 bunch Mint
- inch Fresh root turmeric

Directions:

1. First of all, cut the cauliflower into smaller florets and blend in a food processor or blender.
2. Process until it begins to look like rice.
3. Next, prep the veggies. Roughly chop off the herbs like parsley, mint, and coriander.
4. Throw away the parsley and mint stems but keep that off the coriander.
5. Slice the courgette and kale thinly.
6. Peel off the turmeric and ginger, then grate both into a pan containing coconut oil.
7. Once it begins to get warm, stir the mint, parsley and coriander and coriander stem into the mix.
8. Wait for thirty seconds and stir in the kale and cauliflower.
9. After two to three minutes, add the tamari, spring onions and the remaining herbs.
10. Stir properly and turn off the heat.

11. Lastly, chop the almonds, stir through. Season to taste and sprinkle lime.

Alkaline Salad With Mint And Lemon Toppings

Ingredients:

- Avocado (sliced)
- 3 Asparagus
- 1 bunch Flat leaf parsley
- 2 Courgette (zucchini)
- 220 g Green peas
- 5 Radish
- 1 bunch Cilantro

For The Dressing:

- 1 Garlic clove
- 200 ml Olive oil
- Black pepper and Himalayan salt to taste
- 1/2 bunch Mint
- 2 Shallots
- 3 Lemons
- 20 g Dijon Mustard

Directions:

1. First of all, let's start with the asparagus.
2. Boil water in a pan, when it gets to the boiling point, immerse the asparagus inside, for about one minute.
3. Remove it and rinse immediately in cold water.
4. After that, slice it in long strips. Next, get a frying pan and fry the Zucchini over medium heat until it begins to turn brown.
5. Get a large bowl, mix the cilantro, radish, parsley, peas, avocado, asparagus and zucchini.
6. In other to make the dressing, blend all Ingredients: in a food processor.
7. Finally, dress and season.

Alkaline Sushi-Roll Ups

Ingredients:

For Hummus:

- 1 pinch Cumin
- 1 pinch Himalayan salt
- A glug Olive oil
- 1 tsp Tahini
- 120 g Chickpeas
- 1 Clove of garlic
- 1 Lemon juice
- Almonds handful

For The Roll-Ups:

- 1 Capsicum
- 1 small Coriander/cilantro
- 1 Avocado
- 1 Cucumber
- 2 Zucchini/Courgette
- 1 Carrot

Directions:

For the Hummus:

1. All you have to do is to get a food processor or blender.
2. Blend until everything is smooth.
3. Then add some more lemon or olive oil to suit your taste.

For the Alkaline Sushi Roll-Ups:

1. Cut off both ends of the Zucchini Use a vegetable peeler to peel it into thin, long strips
2. Lay out the zucchini strip and spread the almond hummus on it
3. Add some matchsticks of avocado, veggies and a few pieces of coriander.
4. Spray some of the sesame seeds on top. Roll and enjoy

Artichoke Sauce Ala Quinoa Pasta

Ingredients:

- 3 tablespoons of fresh basil
- 1 a teaspoon of yeast free vegetable stock
- 3 tablespoons of fresh basil
- 1 a teaspoon of organic sea salt
- 1 pinch of cayenne pepper
- 2 tablespoon of cold pressed extra virgin olive oil
- 7 ounce or 220 g spelled pasta
- 8 ounce or 240 g of frozen artichoke
- 5 ounces of fresh tomatoes
- 1 medium sized onion
- 1 clove of garlic
- 1 ounce of pine nuts
- 1 teaspoon of yeast free vegetable stock

Directions:

1. Prepare your Artichokes by cooking them gently until they show a tender texture

2. Cook the pasta to Al Dente following the instructions on your packet

3. Take out your tomatoes and cut them up into cubes

4. Chop up the onions, garlic, and basil into bite sized portions

5. Take a pan and add 2 tablespoons of olive oil over medium heat

6. Add pine nuts, garlic, and onion and stir them for a few minutes

7. Take another bowl and add 1 a cup of water and dissolve yeast free veggie stock

8. Add the mixture to the pan.

9. Simmer it over low heat and keep stirring it for 2 minutes

10. Once done, add basil and season with cayenne pepper and salt

11. Pour the sauce over your pasta. Serve!

Special Pasta Ala Pepper And Tomato Sauce

Ingredients:

- 1 piece of onion
- 2 pieces of garlic cloves
- 1 piece of chili
- 5 pieces of fresh basil leaves
- 2-3 tablespoon of cold pressed olive oil
- Sea salt as needed
- Pepper as needed
- 520 g of vegetable pasta
- 320 g of tomatoes
- 1 a cup of sun-dried tomatoes
- 1 small sized red bell pepper
- 1 small sized Zucchini

Directions:

1. Cook the pasta properly according to the specified package instructions.

2. Cut up the tomatoes, bell pepper, zucchini into fine cubes and chop the chili, garlic, and onions.

3. Take a pan and place it over medium heat

4. Add oil and heat up the oil. Add onions, chili, pepper, and garlic and fry them for a few minutes

5. Add tomatoes, zucchini and cook for 5-10 minutes more. Add basil]

6. Season with pepper and salt to adjust the flavor

7. Add pasta on top your serving plate

8. Pour the sauce and season Serve!